DASH DIET

A Beginner's Guide to Lose Weight, Lower Blood Pressure and Boost Metabolism with Delicious Recipes the Fast and Easy Way

Sandra Rossi

Disclaimer

Any and all information contained herein is not intended to take the place of medical advice from a healthcare professional. This information is for educational and informational purposes only. Readers should always consult with a physician before taking any actions of any kind relating to their health. The author nor publisher will in no way be held responsible for any reader who fails to do so. Any action taken based on these contents is at the sole discretion and liability of the reader.

Published by Sandra Rossi, 1362 E. Main St. #56 El Cajon, CA 92021

First Printing, 2013

ISBN-13: 978-1492824732

ISBN-10: 1492824739

Printed in the United States of America

"The greatest miracle on Earth is the human body. It is stronger and wiser than you may realize, and improving its ability to self-heal is within your control"

Dr Fabrizio Mancini

DEDICATION

To you, the Creator of the Heavens and the Earth.

To my sons, Andrew, Michael and Steven.

To you, the reader.

Table of Contents

Introduction

Are you ready to wake up every morning feeling wonderful? Are you tired of diets that just won't work? Are you tired of feeling weighed down by all the extra weight you have packed on?

In the past twenty years the rate of obesity in America has gradually been on the rise. People all around you battle with hypertension, heart disease, diabetes and numerous other health related issues. We spend millions of dollars every year on medicines that are supposed to help us maintain wellness. Shouldn't there be an easier way? Shouldn't we be able to see results within weeks instead of months and years? Well now there is a way!

Diets are a dime a dozen. If you have seen one diet you have seen them all, but that is not true. The Dash diet is a new diet that has changed the whole structure of dieting. It takes a different approach to eating and makes the food work for you. Participants of this diet have reported lower levels of hypertension and this diet has beneficial qualities for people suffering from Type 2 diabetes. Participants of this diet have started seeing results as soon as two weeks after starting the Dash diet.

DASH DIET: A Beginner's Guide to Lose Weight, Lower Blood Pressure and Boost Metabolism with Delicious Recipes the Fast and Easy Way is a complete comprehensive guide to everything that you need to know about the Dash diet. Included in this guide is an overview of the diet in whole along with the research behind the diet and numerous tips for success and benefits. You will be taken through every part of the diet and be introduced to it in a way that you do not get out of other diets. There are many added bonuses, such as a seven day menu plan and recipes to help get you started on the road to a better you.

This diet is all natural. There are no added diet pills or protein shakes. This diet will take you through how to prepare and eat everyday foods in a way that is more beneficial to your body.

What are you waiting for? Are you ready to take that first step towards a better you?

What is The Dash Diet?

There have been many diets created over the years to help in the battle against obesity. The Dash diet is one among many. However, the Dash diet did not start out as a diet to combat obesity; instead it was formulated to combat high blood pressure or hypertension. The Dash diet stands for:

- D-Dietary

- A-Approach to

- S-Stop

- H-Hypertension

The Dash diet is intended to be a potentially lifelong approach to eating healthier with the added benefit of lowering your blood pressure and preventing hypertension. The diet works with a person on reducing things such as sodium in everyday diets. It also teaches dieters how to eat a variety of different foods that are rich in nutrients that will lower blood pressure and help combat other illnesses such as heart disease, obesity, stroke, diabetes, and osteoporosis. The Dash diet was not developed to be a weight loss program but most people who apply this diet to their everyday lives find that they are able to shed unwanted weight because of the eating guides outlined in this program. The Dash diet emphasizes things like portion control, getting the right amount, the correct nutrients, and eating a variety of healthier foods.

Why was the Dash Diet Created?

Hypertension is one of the greatest health concerns in the United States. High blood pressure puts a person at a higher risk of heart attack, stroke, kidney disease, and heart failure. Obesity is one of the largest contributors to high blood pressure. With these rates steadily on the increase, it was important for scientists to discover a correlation between healthy dieting and incidents of obesity and hypertension. The goal was to discover what types of foods a person could eat that would decrease their likelihood of blood pressure related issues. It was uncovered that eating patterns did affect things like hypertension and so the Dash diet was created.

The Dash Diet: The Research behind the Phenomenon

As you know, the Dash diet is a relatively new eating plan that has revolutionized the way people eat. It boasts impressive health benefits: the diet works to help a person learn better portion control and to lower sodium intake while teaching them the right kinds of food to eat. The Dash diet has been established as a model eating plan and has all of the medical community raving about it. Now the real question is, how did this revolutionary diet come to be?

The Dash Study

The Dash diet started out as a way to battle hypertension or high blood pressure. Blood pressure is the force needed to push blood through the arteries while the heart pumps out the blood. High blood pressure affects millions of people, and the worst part is that most people do not even know that they have it. The research started as a way to study the effects that dieting had on high blood pressure and how different approaches to dieting could correlate with blood pressure. The research found that diet does, in fact, play a role in a person developing high blood pressure; it was also shown that the diets play a role in reducing the risk of high blood pressure.

The National Institute of Health (NIH) created and funded the research. The National Heart, Lung and Blood Institute (NHLBI) directed the studies with the help of five different medical academies in the United States. They were Brigham and Women's Hospital, Johns Hopkins University, Kaiser Permanente

Center for Health Research, Pennington Biomedical Research Center and Duke University Medical Center.

The study took 459 subjects all with normal to high blood pressure, with 27% presenting hypertension. The subjects included both men and women of White and African-American origin. All the subjects averaged around the age of 45. The original group was composed of 2/3 of people of African-American descent because past studies showed that African-Americans have a higher disposition to hypertension (Dash Dieting Eating Plans, 2013).

Every participant was randomly given one of three different diets to follow:

- A normal diet that you would expect a typical American to eat

- A diet with a higher intake of fruits and vegetables

- The Dash diet

The subjects were limited to 1-2 alcoholic beverages a week and mandated to consume around 3,000 mg of sodium each day: 3,000 mg of sodium is roughly equivalent to 1 ¼ teaspoon of table salt. These numbers sound alarming but 3,000 mg of sodium is about 20% below the normal sodium intake for adults (National Heart, 1998,2006).

Within two weeks of starting the trial, the research showed that the subjects following both the Dash diet and the diet that involved more fruit and vegetable intake had reduced their blood pressure. The Dash diet showed greater instances of lower blood pressure, especially with the subjects that began the study already having hypertension. African-Americans who participated in the study were shown to be more sensitive to the dietary changes and experienced more substantial blood pressure reductions. The results were so drastic that they paralleled the results of taking a prescribed medicine for blood pressure.

With these great results the Dash study was followed up with a second study called Dash-Sodium (Dash Dieting Eating Plans, 2013). Scientists wanted to better understand the relationship between sodium and blood pressure. The study involved 412 new participants, except this time 41% had hypertension. The subjects were randomly chosen and assigned to either a typical diet or the Dash diet. Within both groups the subjects were mandated to follow three different sodium levels:

- High sodium= 3,300 mg per day

- Intermediate sodium= 2,400-3,300 mg per day

- Low sodium= 1,500 mg or less per day

In both test groups, the research showed lowered blood pressure in both groups who were required to reduce their sodium levels. The data showed that the lower the sodium level, the lower the blood pressure tended to be. The group that saw the largest decline of blood pressure and hypertension were the subjects following the Dash diet at its lowest level of sodium intake. It also showed that blood pressure was lower on the Dash eating plan regardless of which sodium levels. The subjects that had already presented with hypertension at the beginning of the studies showed significant decreases in blood pressure. This study concluded that lowered sodium levels in every diet were directly correlated with lowering blood pressure (National Heart, 1998,2006).

How the Final Diet was decided

While the studies were being conducted scientists discovered that lowered blood pressure also contributed to lower levels in fats, especially saturated, and cholesterol. They wanted to develop the diet in a well-rounded way that would ensure the participant received the most out of all the other nutrients in the diet. They found the perfect balance by including whole grains, poultry, fish, and decreased amounts of high fat dairy products. The diet reduces levels of red meats, certain fats such as saturated fats, and foods with high sugar content. They formulated the Dash diet to be high in potassium, magnesium, and calcium. All of these different nutrients have also been found to help win the war against blood pressure. Foods with the best level of these specific nutrients were:

- Fruits

- Nuts

- Vegetables

- Beans

- Seeds

- Low-fat diary

The Dash diet may have been created with the benefits of lowering blood pressure, but the truth is the Dash diet aids everyone.

The Benefits of the Dash Diet

The Dietary Approach to Stop Hypertension, or Dash diet, allows participants to lower their blood pressure in a safe and natural way. The diet takes a low sodium approach to dieting along with greater portion control and learning to eat the foods that are good for the body.

While the Dash diet was originally intended with a significant purpose in mind, it has been found that it comes along with a list of potential health benefits.

Benefit One- Lower Blood Pressure

As stated before, your blood pressure is the force needed to push blood through all the veins and arteries of the body. Blood pressure is dependent on many different factors such as the strength of a person's heartbeat, a person's overall health, age, elasticity of the arterial walls, and the thickness of the blood. The higher a person's blood pressure, the harder the heart has to work in order to continue to pump the appropriate amount of blood through the veins in the body.

Dieting plays a big part in the role of lowering a person's blood pressure. With the Dash diet's different approach to lowering sodium and upping the amounts of potassium, calcium, and magnesium, all nutrients that help with lowering blood pressure, the diet is especially beneficial to lowering blood pressure.

As mentioned before, the higher the blood pressure, the harder the heart has to work to keep the appropriate amount of blood flowing through the body. High blood pressure also opens the body up to numerous other diseases and disorders. Lowering a person's blood pressure is one of the most efficient ways to prevent other disorders from occurring.

Benefit Two- Weight Loss

Maintaining a healthy weight is one of the most important health advantages a person can have. Obesity is a growing epidemic in America and many other countries around the world. People who are overweight or obese have higher instances of problems such as heart disease, high blood pressure, and numerous other potentially life threatening illnesses.   Even though the Dash diet was not created to stimulate weight loss, it has been found to be an overall effective weight loss plan. The Dash diet takes a dietary approach that reduces sodium, cholesterol, and fats (especially saturated fats). The original Dash diet is based on a normal 2,000 calorie per day diet. A person wishing to lose weight would just need to adjust the calorie intake so that they would only consume around 1,500 calories per day.

Benefit Three- Faster Metabolism

Metabolism is a very complex system of different enzymes, and hormones that work together to convert the food a person consumes into fuel, and also affects how well a person's body burns that fuel. Metabolism is usually thought of as the rate a person burns calories and how quickly a person gains or loses weight. There are many different factors that contribute to the efficiency of a person's metabolism.

People who are obese tend to have higher metabolisms because their bodies have to work so much harder. When starting this diet, due to already high metabolism rates, it will be easier for a heavier person to lose weight more rapidly than average. Also many of the different foods that the Dash diet encourages a person to eat such as, apples, low fat yogurts, celery, lean meats and fish, beans, all work to raise your metabolism.

Benefit Four-Heart Disease

It is widely known that people who eat healthier, lower sodium levels, and exercise regularly will have a much better chance of fighting off heart disease than other people who do not. One of the reasons this diet works so well to combat heart disease is that it helps eliminate one of the leading causes of heart disease: hypertension. Cholesterol contributes to a lot of artery blockage found around the heart. The Dash diet helps to lower cholesterol levels, which in turn lowers the risk heart disease caused by blockage. In recent studies it has been found that women who follow the Dash diet have a significantly lower rate for the instances of heart disease (Kelli Miller, 2008).

Benefit Five-Bone Health

Osteoporosis is a bone disease that causes bones to become more fragile and more likely to break or fracture. We normally perceive this as an "old person's disease," but that is not the case anymore. Osteoporosis and other bone diseases can occur at any age. Poor bone health can be attributed to not getting enough of the proper nutrients to sustain bone health.

People who have had long term use of the Dash diet have seen significant results in the reduction of bone turnover; this could be attributed to the higher levels of potassium, calcium, and magnesium a person consumes on the Dash diet.

Benefit Six- Managing Diabetes Type 2

Diabetes is where a person's body has problems processing insulin. It is normally referred to as insulin resistance or hyperglycemia. Type 2 diabetes means the pancreas cannot keep up with the levels of insulin needed to keep the blood glucose levels at normal. Type 2 diabetes has been found to be the most common instance of diabetes.

Being obese is one of the largest risk factors for people with type 2 diabetes. Though the Dash diet was not designed with weight loss in mind, it has been proven that if followed correctly at a lower calorie intake, the participant can in fact lose weight. This is the first important step in preventing instances of Type 2 diabetes. The Dash diet is uniquely planned to ensure that sugars and additional fats are phased out or greatly reduced. It also is developed to provide participants with the appropriate nutritional values that they need to maintain a healthy body system. The Dash diet is also lower in starch, which is the enemy of many participants with diabetes. Weight loss has also been thought to contribute to better insulin sensitivity, which allows insulin to go in and get its job done by burning more energy (John A. Tayek, 2002).

Benefit Seven- A Better You

This is probably the best benefit any diet such as the Dash diet can provide for a person. The Dash diet teaches the dieters how to do portion control, and which foods are good and which are bad for them. It helps participants lower their blood pressure and help to ensure that the pressure stays down. The Dash diet caters to those who wish to lose weight by allowing for calorie cuts and adjusting the serving sizes accordingly. It helps people suffering from Type 2 diabetes in helping lower their levels and to hopefully become independent of medications. The best benefit is that it improves a person's overall health, and once better health has been achieved, a person is one step closer to living longer and having a wonderful quality of life.

What Can a Person Eat in the Dash Diet?

Sodium amounts and calories permitted

Regardless of which sodium plan a person chooses, either 1500 mg or 2300 mg of sodium per day, all the food choices are the same. The goal of the Dash diet is to lower sodium and to teach the participants a healthier way of eating less sodium, fats, and cholesterol. You can chose a diet anywhere from 1500- 3000 calories per day. The following are the recommended servings per day for a 2,000 calorie diet:

- **6-8 servings of grains a day**: This includes bread, cereal, pastas, and rice. Whole grains are preferred because they are more fibrous and packed full of more nutrients than normal grains; they are also lower in overall fat. Great examples of grain are: whole grain bagels, whole grain bread, whole grain pasta, English muffin, pita bread, oatmeal and brown rice. Bad grains include: salted pretzels and saltine crackers.

- **4-5 servings of vegetables a day**: Every diet known to man emphasizes the importance of regular vegetable intake. There are a large variety of different vegetables to choose from. Vegetables as a side dish are overrated: there are so many creative ways to incorporate vegetables into the main attraction of any meal. Fresh or frozen vegetables are always the better choices. However, if a person has to buy canned vegetables, they should take into consideration the label information and make sure to choose low sodium or no salt added canned vegetable. Examples of good vegetables are: carrots, celery, cauliflower, tomatoes, collard greens, potatoes, sweet potatoes and kale.

Examples of not good vegetables are: canned vegetables with high sodium levels, pickled vegetables, and vegetables cooked in some sort of fat or fried.

- **4-5 servings of fruits a day**: Fruit is the ultimate snack food. It is packed full of fiber, magnesium, and potassium and low in fat. Fruit is one of the most versatile foods a person will find. It can be any meal, snack, or dessert. If the peel is edible leave it on. Fresh or frozen fruit is always the better route to go, but canned fruit will do as long as it has no sugar added. Good fruit examples are: strawberries, bananas, apples, apricots, grapefruit, oranges and kiwi. Fruits that are not allowed are fruits canned in sugary syrup.

- **2-3 servings of dairy products a day**: It is no secret that dairy products are rich in calcium, protein, and numerous vitamins. The key is to pick products that are low fat or fat free, otherwise dairy products are large sources of mainly saturated fats. Take into consideration how much sodium each dairy product contains. There are a small number of people who have trouble digesting dairy products so it is okay to substitute lactose free products in order to obtain the dairy quota. When substituting, it is important to get the lactose free products and not substitute with soy or other alternatives, as the results would not work the same. Examples of approved dairy products are: 1% milk, low fat cottage cheese, and fat free yogurt. Bad examples would be: basically any full fat dairy product.

- **2 servings of lean meats, chicken, or fish a day**: Meats of all kinds are rich sources of protein and numerous vitamins; they also carry a large variety of fats and cholesterol. This is a big area where portion control comes into play. A serving size of meat in this category is roughly around 3 ounces. While using this diet a person should never fry their meat; they should instead choose to bake, grill, or roast the meat. Also, choose lean cuts of meat, like "loin" or "round cuts".

In this category fish win out on overall health benefits because they are chock-full of omega -3 and help to naturally lower a person's cholesterol. Eggs are allowed but no more than four per week. Good examples of the lean meats are: halibut, cod, venison, salmon, and no fat pork or lamb. Examples of bad meats would be: any meat that is smoked or especially salty such as bacon and sausage.

- **4-5 servings of nuts/seeds/legumes per week**: These are all great sources of protein and numerous other health benefits. This is also where soy-based foods and meat alternatives are taken into consideration. While different nuts are high in fat content, the benefits they provide outweigh the additional fat. Good examples from this food group are: almonds, hazelnuts, peanuts, walnuts, mixed nuts, beans, split peas and lentils. Try to avoid nuts covered in salt because they are higher in sodium.

- **2-3 servings fat/oil a day**: The body needs fat to be able to appropriately absorb vitamins and nutrients. In order to maintain a healthy immune system it is important to consume a decent amount of the right fats. This is where light salad dressing and soft margarine come into play. With so few servings a day, this is another area where portion control comes in handy. When used in moderation good fats/oils are: olive oil, canola oil, low fat cream cheese, low-fat mayonnaise and avocados. Bad fat/ oils are: high sodium gravies and peanut oil.

- **5 servings of sweets a week**: Yes, the Dash diet does not make a person forsake sweets; they should just be low in fat. Just like any diet, portion control is important, and a bit of self-control is essential. With moderation and portion control approved sweets are: hard candy, maple syrup, fruit punch, fruit flavored gelatin, sorbet, ices, jams and jellies. It is probably not a good idea to have that slice of chocolate cake. Again, moderation is the key in this category but for a better choice you can eat raisins, dates or figs.

- **Alcohol**- To get the most out of the Dash diet a dieter should not consume more than two drinks if they are a man and no more than one drink if they are a woman per day (Clinic, 2013).

Eating healthy can be difficult. The Dash diet, even though it was not created with weight loss in mind, provides a structured plan in order to better obtain weight loss goals.

Getting Started on the Dash Diet

You have finally done it! You have finally taken the initiative to better yourself. You know that one of the biggest things that you have to do is to work on your health. After all, better health means a better you. You have done all the research that is available to you about the Dash diet and you have decided that it is time to get started. That is the exact moment that you stop and wonder how in the world do I get started?

Commitment and Motivation

Getting started is easier than you think. The very first thing you have to do is commit to the idea. This is the most important part of the whole 'better you' process. A diet is only as efficient as the dieter's will to succeed; so unless you are ready to fully commit to the idea, you will not be ready to get started. Motivation is the best friend to commitment. You can use different motivators such as an awesome new dress or an expensive pair of feel-good shoes to motivate yourself to do almost anything. Motivation is another key to successful dieting.

Figure out Where You Are At

The next step is, knowing your facts. Professionals use a person's body mass index (BMI) or their basal metabolic rate (BMR) to determine the classification a person falls into.

The body mass index is an equation that takes into consideration the amount you weigh and how tall you are. Obesity is defined when a person's body mass index exceeds 30. Below is the equation used to calculate your own BMI:

$$108K$$

$$BMI = \frac{\text{Weigt in pounds} \times 703}{\text{Height in Inches} \times \text{Height in Inches}} \quad = 30$$

$$3600$$

http://www.nhlbi.nih.gov/guidelines/obesity/bmi_tbl.htm

Your basal metabolic rate (BMR) is the energy (in calories) used by your body at rest to maintain normal body functions such as keeping your heart pumping, your lungs working to process oxygen, and your brain running. There are many different factors that can influence your BMR, such as your age, gender, height, and exercising habits. To calculate your BMR you have to go through a bit more than you would for your BMI.

Do not panic! You do not have to be a mathematician to understand these formulas. Besides, if all else fails, there are plenty of really reliable online BMI and BMR calculating tools. One of the easiest equations to calculate your BMR is the Mifflin Equation:

Men
10 x weight (kg)[i] + 6.25 x height (cm)[ii] - 5 x age (y) + 5

Women
10 x weight (kg) + 6.25 x height (cm) - 5 x age (y) - 161.

The reason some people prefer using the BMR is because your BMR can tell you how many calories your body needs to consume in order to maintain your current weight or in this case how many calories are too many calories.

Visit the Doctor

Now that you have a general idea of your body, it is time to head to your friendly neighborhood doctor. This is such an important step that a lot of people skip. Unless you have a degree in biology, chemistry, or nutrition you probably have no real idea how your body runs and the appropriate amounts of nutrition needed to sustain wellness. This is where your doctor comes in. A doctor can take in all the information that you have gathered and help you to formulate the best exercise and eating plans so that you can lose weight without risking harm to yourself. It is also important to go consult with a doctor in the event that you have a disease or a family history of diseases such as high blood pressure, diabetes, or heart disease, in order to be monitored more specifically. Who knows, maybe your results will help your doctor prescribe the Dash diet to someone else in need.

Get Your House Ready

Once you have obtained your doctor's blessing it is important to go through your house and get rid of all the processed fatty foods that will tempt you to stray from dieting. You don't have to throw them away, but you need to get them out of your eyesight. Go around your neighborhood or to less privileged neighborhoods and donate the boxes of extra food to people in need. They will appreciate the food and it will allow you to start your diet with a clean slate. Yes, this means all of your secret stashes of snacks have got to go. Don't try to deny that you have a secret stash of snacks; we all do and we all secretly eat chocolates in the corner while no one is looking.

This is a great time to put your research skills to work. You need to start looking for awesome recipes that will help you make healthy meals without having to sacrifice taste. It is also a good idea to locate some local farms or farmer markets that will be able to provide fresher produce choices. If the area you live in does not have these options that is fine. Most of the supermarkets have everything that you need to maintain your dietary guidelines. Just always be conscious of labels, and make sure that you always keep an eye on the sugar and sodium levels of every piece of food that you pick up to take home with you.

Exercise

Now here is the hard part, you have to exercise. There is no such thing as a miracle diet that can help you reach your goal weight without a little extra work put into it. If there was then everyone would be skinny. Exercising does not have to be evil. If you think of exercising as every time you move, instead of sectioning off certain things like walking twenty minutes or running around the track, you will find it much easier. If you need to walk for twenty minutes, go to the store and browse through different areas. Any shopper knows that at large supermarkets you walk everywhere, and half the time you have to go across the store half a dozen times because you forgot something. You can vary the speed in which you walk. If you have problems with being able to deny yourself, steer clear of the food aisles and instead go through the clothes aisle and pick out a new skinny outfit that you will buy after you hit your target weight. If you are feeling adventurous you can go out to the swimming pool or go out for a brisk run in the park. Bicycling is also a wonderful way to get in the extra exercise that you need and burn lots of calories. You can plan a hike in the woods with friends to help keep you motivated. There are a million other ways to exercise, you just have to find the right one that works for you.

If you are having a rough day, clean something. It is exercise: sweeping or mopping floors or stretching up high to get that dust off the fan blades. If that does not work, go to the store and purchase a new work out outfit. You will immediately feel better about working out if you have an appealing outfit and a comfortable pair of shoes to wear.

Keep Positive

Remember that at the very beginning it will be hard. Your body is not used to being denied that slice of chocolate cake or doing the extra exercise that you have started to incorporate into your daily routine. There is no shame in falling off the wagon every once in a while, it is not a failure unless you give up trying. You have to take every day as a new challenge and head into it with that mindset.

A wonderful way to keep on track is to have a diet buddy to hold you accountable. This buddy will be dieting with you as well, so you work as a support system to keep each other in check. If you do not have a buddy available, then do things such as keeping a list of all the bad foods that you should avoid. If you see a reminder of the foods that you should not buy it will stick in your mind better. It is important to utilize a menu plan: a menu plan is where you plan all of your meals and your snacks ahead of time. This will help you to not stray off the path. It is also a secret comfort; if you have a menu plan in place you are never stuck wondering what you are going to make for dinner, therefore it is less likely that you will mess up your dieting.

Resources

You need to utilize all the resources available to you. If there is a gym close by go and use their equipment. If there is a local park go there for your walks. There are even exercise classes in certain communities that you can go to for free that are filled with other people who are working on losing weight and can share their stories and support. The internet is also full of different resources such as:

http://www.dashdietoregon.org/

www.dietaryguidelines.gov

http://healthyeating.nhlbi.nih.gov/

http://www.nih.gov/

to name a few that provide more information about the Dash diet and also offer resources such as recipes and meal plans.

Dieting is easier now than it has ever been. Are you ready to take that first step?

Examples of Dash Diet Foods and their Portion Sizes

By now we all know how important portion control is. The Dash diet is full of really great serving selections that you have to eat every day, but how are you supposed to know what serving size is too big. Recipes will only tell you so much, and it is important when making meal plans to know the portions that you are allowed to eat. These are examples of what **one serving** would be. Use this as a guide:

Grains

1 slice whole-wheat bread
1 oz. dry cereal
1/2 cup cooked cereal
1/2 cup cooked rice or pasta

Vegetables

1 cup raw leafy green vegetable
1/2 cup cut-up raw or cooked vegetables
6 fluid oz. low-sodium vegetable juice

Fruits

1 medium fruit
1/4 cup dried fruit
1/2 cup fresh, frozen or canned fruit
6 fluid oz. 100% fruit juice

Low- fat or Nonfat Dairy Products

1 cup (8 fluid oz.) milk
1 cup yogurt
1 1/2 oz. of cheese

Lean Meats, Poultry, Eggs and Fish

1 oz. cooked lean meat, skinless poultry or fish
1 egg (no more than 4 a week)
2 egg whites

Nuts, seeds and legumes

1/3 cup (1.5 oz.) nuts
2 tablespoons peanut butter
2 tablespoons (1/2 oz.) seeds
1/2 cup cooked legumes (dried beans or peas)

Fats and oils

1 teaspoon soft margarine
1 teaspoon of vegetable oil
1 tablespoon low- fat mayonnaise
1 tablespoon of regular salad dressing
2 tablespoon of low fat salad dressing

Sweets and added sugars

1 tablespoon sugar
1 tablespoon jelly or jam
1/2 cup sorbet
1 cup (8 fluid oz.) sugar-sweetened lemonade

http://www.nhlbi.nih.gov/health/prof/heart/other/chdblack/aa_manual/session6.htm#serving

Delicious Recipes the Fast and Easy Way

We all are no strangers to dieting at this point, but like with every new diet, you have to find recipes that work for you and your lifestyle. Below are a few recipes compiled together that adhere to the strict guidelines that the Dash diet is all about. You can eat the recipes at any meal.

These are just examples of recipes that can be implemented in your diet. There are a lot of resources from where you can get more, the internet, books, magazines, your family, your friends to name a few.

Breakfast Recipes

Almond Butter Blueberries and Banana Smoothie

This is a great recipe to start your day, easy to make and will keep you full for at least two or three hours.

Serves: 1

Nutritional tip:

This recipe is full of potassium and antioxidants, nutrients to help you control your blood pressure.

Ingredients:

1 cup of fat-free milk
1 tablespoon of almond butter (all natural)
1 fresh or frozen medium banana
½ cup of blueberries

Preparation:

Put all the ingredients together in a blender, then blend them until they become very smooth, if it is too thick add 1 ½ oz. of cold water.

Nutritional Information:

Per serving: 385 calories, 20 g protein, 63 g carbohydrates, 9 g total fat, 6 g fiber, 190 mg sodium

Applesauce French Toast

Get fueled in the morning with this tasty French toast.

Serves: 6

Nutritional tip:

To make this recipe a full meal, try to add a glass of non-fat milk.

Ingredients:

2 eggs
2/3 cup of non-fat milk
¼ tsp.[iii] of ground cinnamon
¼ cup of applesauce
6 slice of whole wheat bread
1 tsp. of vanilla extract
1 tbsp.[iv] of maple syrup

Preparation:

1. In a bowl, beat eggs, non-fat milk, cinnamon, applesauce and vanilla extract.
2. Soak each slice of bread in the mixture.
3. Cook on greased skillet over medium heat until both sides become golden brown.
4. Serve with blueberries and strawberries for the topping and maple syrup over it.
5. Serve it hot!

Nutritional Information:

Serving Size: 1 slice

Per serving: 250 calories, 8 g protein, 28 g carbohydrates, 3 g fat, 2 g fiber, 210 mg sodium

Vegetables and Cheese Egg Muffin Omelets

You can enjoy an omelet for breakfast and still be eating healthy. This recipe would be good to prepare ahead of time so that way you will have it ready every day of the week. You are to choose the vegetables you like the most, never be afraid to experiment with different vegetable combinations.

Serves: 9

Nutritional tip:

To have a complete well-balanced and tasty breakfast, you can add a fruit salad, glass of low-fat milk and whole wheat toast.

Ingredients:

1 cup of red peppers (diced)
1 cup of mushrooms (diced)
1 cup of spinach (diced)
1 cup of onions (diced)
4 whole eggs
1 cup of egg whites
¼ cup of low-fat cheddar
¼ cup of parmesan cheese
1 tablespoon of olive oil
¼ tsp. of low sodium salt
¼ tsp. of pepper

Preparation:

1. Preheat oven to 350° F.

2. Put all the vegetables in a bowl and add the olive oil, low sodium salt and pepper, toss together.

3. In a greased muffin tin, pour the vegetables in each muffin hole.

4. In a separate bowl add the grated parmesan cheese, eggs, and egg whites and beat them together.

5. Pour the mixture over the vegetables up to a little over ¾ full.

6. Add the low fat cheddar on top of the mixture, and bake it for 20 minutes.

7. Put the muffin omelets in Ziploc bags and refrigerate them.

Nutritional Information:

Serving Size: 1 mini-omelet

Per serving: 104 calories, 9 g protein, 3 g carbohydrates, 7 g total fat, 213 mg sodium

Oatmeal Waffles/or Pancakes

Delicious pancakes for breakfast are the best choice for everyone.

Serves: 4

Nutritional tip:

This recipe is a complete meal by itself. You can add half a glass of non-fat milk or some fruit juice of your choice.

Ingredients:

For the fruit topping:

2 cups of frozen or fresh strawberries, rinsed, stems removed, and cut in half
1 cup of frozen or fresh blackberries, rinsed
2 cups of frozen or fresh blueberries
1 tsp. of maple syrup

For waffles:

1 cup of whole wheat flour
1/2 cup of oats
2 tsp. of baking powder
1 tsp. of maple syrup
1/4 cup of chopped pecans (unsalted)
2 large eggs, separated (for pancakes see the notes below)
1 ½ cup of non-fat milk
1 tbsp. of vegetable oil

Preparation:

1. Preheat the waffle iron.
2. Grab a large bowl and mix together the oats, flour, maple syrup, baking powder and pecans.
3. In another bowl, mix the egg yolks, non-fat milk and vegetable oil well.
4. Add the liquid mixture to the dry ingredients in the large bowl, stir together and make sure not to mix too much because mixture should be a little bit lumpy.
5. Whip the egg whites to medium peaks then fold the egg whites gently into batter (for pancakes, see below).
6. Pour batter into the preheated waffles iron, cook until the steam stops coming out of the iron (or if the signal shows that it is done) the perfect waffle should be crisp and well-browned on the outside with a moist, light feeling coming out of the iron. (For the pancakes, decline this step and just cook the pancakes).
7. For serving, add light dusting powdered sugar and some fresh fruit to each waffle.

Tips for pancakes:

Do not separate the eggs. Mix the non-fat milk with whole eggs and oil, and eliminate steps 4 and 5.

Nutritional Information:

Serving size: 6 inch waffle
Per serving: 340 calories, 14 g protein, 50 g carbohydrates, 11 g total fat, 9 g total fiber, 331 mg sodium

Lunch Recipes

Non-mayo Tuna Salad

This recipe has the same taste as the traditional mayonnaise tuna salad.

Serves: 2

Nutritional tip:

This is a tasty tuna salad that has less than 200 mg of sodium per serving. You can substitute the spinach for arugula or mixed greens if you want. Try this recipe with different shapes of whole wheat pasta like shell or bowtie. Serve this dish with a cup of low-sodium soup, a glass of non-fat milk and a piece of fruit for a complete meal.

Ingredients:

5 oz.ᵛ of light tuna, canned in water and drained
1 tbsp. of extra virgin olive oil
1 tsp. of red wine vinegar
¼ cup of green onion tops, chopped
2 cups of arugula
1 cup of whole wheat pasta
1 tbsp. of fresh parmesan cheese

Preparation:

1. In a large bowl toss tuna with olive oil, vinegar, arugula, onion

and cooked whole wheat pasta.

2. Divide the salad into two plates and top each plate with pepper and parmesan.

3. Serve immediately.

Nutritional Information:

Per serving: 245 calories, 23 g protein, 23 g carbohydrates, 7 g total fat, 1 g fiber, 190 mg sodium

Black Bean and Corn Salsa Salad

A delicious and light meal for those days that you don't want to eat too much.

Serves: 8

Nutritional tip:

Beans and crunchy vegetables are the best choice for summer salads. If you are going to use canned beans, make sure to use low-sodium or no salt added.

Ingredients:

Salad:

2 cups of black beans (cooked), or 2 15 oz. cans of drained and rinsed black beans
2 cups of corn kernels
3/4 cup of seeded and chopped red bell pepper
3/4 cup of seeded and chopped orange bell pepper
2 small seeded and minced small jalapeno chilies
3/4 cup of finely chopped sweet white or red onion
1 large ripe tomato (chopped)
1/2 cup of finely chopped fresh parsley or cilantro

Dressing:

1/3 cup of olive oil
¼ cup of lime juice
1 clove garlic
1/3 tsp. of ground cumin

1/3 tsp. of ground coriander

Preparation:

For the dressing:

1. Grab a small bowl and whisk together the lime juice, olive oil, coriander, garlic and cumin until blended.
2. In order to allow the flavors to mix together, leave the mixture aside for 30 minutes.

For the greens:

1. Grab a large bowl and mix the corn, black beans, jalapenos, red and orange bell peppers and onion.
2. Pour the dressing over the salad mixture and toss it smoothly to combine well without crushing the beans, then add the tomatoes and toss the mixture slightly.
3. Cover and keep in the fridge to let the flavors blend. Before serving, make sure to add parsley or cilantro and toss well.

Nutritional Information:

Per serving: 190 calories, 6 g protein, 23 g carbohydrates, 9.5 g total fat, 6 g fiber, 106 mg sodium

Pear, Turkey and Cheese Sandwich

Fresh pear makes the sandwich more tasty and healthy.

Serves: 2

Nutritional tip:

When you shop for lean deli meats, be careful because some are loaded with salt so make sure that the product you buy is low in sodium.

Ingredients:

2 slices of whole grain bread

2 tsp. of Dijon mustard

2 slices of cooked turkey (reduced-sodium)

1 pear, thinly sliced and cored

¼ cup of low-fat mozzarella cheese (shredded)

¼ tsp. of ground pepper

Preparation:

1. On each slice of bread, spread 1 tsp. of mustard.
2. Put one slice of turkey on each slice of the whole grain bread.
3. Put pear slices on the turkey and then add 2 tablespoons of low-fat mozzarella cheese on the top.
4. Sprinkle with pepper.
5. Broil it, it will take about 2 or 3 minutes or until the pears and turkey are warm and also the cheese   melts.
6. When serving, cut each sandwich in half and serve it open-face.

Nutritional Information:

Per serving: 180 calories, 14 g protein, 28 g carbohydrate, 5 g fat,
8 g fiber, 480 mg sodium

Pizza in a Pita Bread

This recipe is like having a real pizza!!

Serves: 2

Nutritional tip:

Add a green salad with vegetables to complete a meal.

Ingredients:

2 pieces of whole wheat pita bread
1/3 cup of low-sodium mozzarella cheese
¼ cup of tomato or pizza sauce
Vegetables: red onion, green onion, red bell pepper, portabella mushrooms

Preparation:

1. Preheat oven to 300 degrees.
2. Open the pita bread, add the pizza sauce and all the vegetables of your choice.
3. Cover the pita with aluminum foil and bake until cheese melts; it will take approximately 5 to 10 minutes.

Nutritional Information:

Per serving: 170 calories, 11 g protein, 24 g carbohydrates, 8 g fat, 4 g fiber, 310 mg sodium

Dinner Recipes

Chicken and Vegetables Stir Fry

Easy to make and well balanced, let us eat Chinese tonight!!!

Serves: 4

Nutritional tip:

To get the most nutrients from your meal and also to limit the added sugar, use 100% fresh orange juice. For a complete meal, add a glass of low-fat milk.

Ingredients:

1/3 cup of orange juice
1 tbsp. of low-sodium soy sauce
1 tbsp. of Schezuan sauce
2 tsp. of cornstarch
1 tbsp. of olive oil
1 lb. of chicken breast, cut in one inch pieces
2 cups of fresh broccoli
1 6-oz. package of peas (frozen)
2 cups of shredded cabbage
2 cups of cooked brown rice
1 tbsp. of sesame seeds (optional)

Preparation:

1. Grab a small bowl and mix the 100% orange juice, low-sodium

soy sauce, cornstarch and Schezuan sauce. Put the mixture aside.
2. Put olive oil in the wok and add the chicken then stir fry until it is done, it will take about 6 minutes.
3. Add the broccoli, snow peas, cabbage and the sauce mixture.
4. Cook the vegetables for five minutes or until they are done.
5. Serve the stir fry with brown rice. You can add some sesame seeds.

Nutritional Information:

Per serving: 340 calories, 28 g protein, 35 g carbohydrates, 8 g total fat, 5 g fiber, 240 mg sodium

Classic Grilled Salmon with Dill Sauce

A classic grilled salmon recipe to enjoy with your friends and family.

Serves: 4

Nutritional tip:

If you are looking for omega-3 fats then salmon is the best choice, because it can lower the risk associated with heart disease. You can add steamed asparagus and brown rice.

Ingredients:

½ cup of low fat mayonnaise
2 tbsp. of fresh dill, minced
1 tsp. of brown sugar
1 tbsp. and 1 tsp. of Dijon mustard
2 tsp. of olive oil
1 lb. of salmon steaks

Preparation:

1. Grab a small bowl, combine the first six ingredients and then put them aside.
2. Spray the racks of the grill with a nonstick cooking spray.
3. Cover the salmon steaks with olive oil and then grill the salmon steaks over for 5 minutes, spread the mayonnaise mixture and continue to grill until is easily flaked.
4. Put the salmon steaks into platter and serve them with brown rice and some vegetables for a complete meal.

Nutritional Information:

Per serving: 218 calories, 26 g protein, 2 g carbohydrates, 11 g total fat, 0 g fiber, 81 mg sodium

Turkey Loaf

Easy dinner for those who want something different!

Serves: 8

Nutritional tip:

You can use the leftovers from this recipe and make sandwiches with some lettuce, tomato and avocado slices. You can add oven-roasted potatoes, green beans and a glass of fat-free milk to have a complete DASH meal.

Ingredients:

1 ½ pounds of lean turkey breast
10 oz. of fresh spinach, chopped
1 cup of uncooked oats
½ cup of carrots, shredded
2 egg whites or 1 egg beaten lightly
1/3 cup of non-fat milk
1 ½ tsp. of Italian seasoning
¼ tsp. of black pepper

Preparation:

1. Preheat oven to 350 degrees.
2. Mix all the ingredients in a large bowl, do not mix thoroughly.
3. Put the mix in a 13x9 inch baking pan.
4. Bake for one hour.
5. Keep it out of oven for 5 minutes before slicing.

Nutritional Information:

Per Serving: 150 calories, 24 g protein, 11 g carbohydrate, 2 g total fat, 3 g fiber, 105 mg sodium

Chicken with Oranges and Avocado

This is a delicious grilled chicken with a beautiful and tasty garnish. This recipe is easy to prepare and a great source of calcium.

Serves: 4

Nutritional Tip:

We are going to marinate the chicken breasts with special ingredients. After finishing, discard the marinade to avoid any contamination with other foods.

Ingredients:

1 cup of low fat yogurt
1/3 cup of chopped red onion
1 tbsp. of chopped cilantro
1 tbsp. of honey
¼ tsp. of low sodium salt
¼ tsp. of ground black pepper
4 chicken breasts - 6 oz. each

Garnish:

1 avocado
1/4 cup of lime juice
2 oranges, peeled and cut in sections
1 small red onion, thinly sliced

Preparation:

1. Mix the first 6 ingredients except the chicken in a large bowl.
2. Add the chicken to the mixture.
3. Cover the bowl and refrigerate for 30 minutes.
4. Preheat the grill or broiler.
5. Remove the chicken from the marinade and discard the marinade.
6. Sprinkle the chicken with salt and pepper.
7. Grill the chicken and cook until the juices run clear.
8. While chicken is cooking, squeeze some lime juice over the avocado and toss it so that it doesn't discolor.
9. Add the oranges, onion and cilantro.
10. Season with salt and serve on top of the chicken.

Nutritional Information:

Per serving: 366 calories, 47 g protein, 19 g carbohydrates, 12 g total fat, 3 g fiber, 265 mg sodium

Dessert Recipes

Yogurt, Blueberries, Almonds and Honey

This is a delicious treat that is very healthy and rich in antioxidants and calcium for your bones. It is sweet and very crunchy!!!

Serves: 4

Nutritional Tip:

You are getting your daily servings of fruits, nuts and dairy with this recipe. Fruits are very sweet by nature so you can have a treat and still be eating very healthy. It is easy to make.

Ingredients:

2 cups of fresh or frozen blueberries
4 teaspoons of honey
4 cups of plain low fat yogurt
4 tablespoons of chopped almonds

Preparation:

1. Place 1 cup of yogurt into each of 4 serving dishes, add ½ cup of blueberries over the yogurt in each of the dishes.

2. Add each with 1 teaspoon of honey and then 1 tablespoon of almonds.

Nutritional Information:

Per Serving: 200 calories, 12 g protein, 30 g carbohydrates, 6 g fat, 4 g fiber, 150 mg sodium

Baked Bananas

You will be surprised how bananas make a delicious dessert.

Serves: 5

Serving size: 1 banana

Nutritional Tip: Make a complete meal by adding 1 glass of low fat milk and a cup of your favorite soup: tomato, avocado soup, creamy mushroom soup to name a few examples. You will love the crunchy nuts!!

Ingredients:

5 bananas, sliced in half
5 tablespoons of brown sugar
3 tablespoons of soft margarine
½ cup of raisins
¼ cup of pecans, cut in little pieces

Directions:

1. Put the sliced bananas in a light greased pan.
2. Cover the bananas with brown sugar, soft margarine, raisins and pecans.
3. Bake at 320 degrees for 25 minutes.
4. Save the rest in the refrigerator.

Nutritional Information:

Per serving: 310 calories, 2 g protein, 52 g carbohydrates, 12 g total fat, 75 mg sodium

Baked Apples and Raisins

This recipe is perfect for those days that you have that sweet craving and want to satisfy it. You can add a glass of low fat milk or almond milk and you will be in heaven!!!

Serves: 2

Nutritional tip:

 Apples and raisins are high in fiber and are full of health benefits, rich in potassium, vitamin A, C and flavonoids and have no fat or sodium. Raisins are a good source of calcium and help you keep the blood clean and flowing.

Ingredients:

2 fresh apples
4 tbsp. of raisins
2 tsp. of brown sugar
2 tsp. of soft margarine
¼ tsp. of cinnamon to taste

Preparation:

1. Rinse the apples and cut the tops and the bottoms of each one.
2. Make a hole in each one and remove the core with the seeds.
3. Place the apples in a baking dish.
4. Sprinkle cinnamon inside the apple and over the top of each one.
5. Fill the center of each apple with raisins until it is full.
6. Cover the top with brown sugar and soft margarine.

7. Bake them for 20 minutes at 300* F or until it is soft.

8. Cool before serving.

Nutritional Information:

Per serving: 235 calories, 1 g protein, 50 g carbohydrates, 4 g fat, 8 g fiber, 20 mg sodium

Refreshing Fruit Salad

The best dessert you can ever have are fruits!!

Serves: 8

Serving size: 2/3 of a cup

Nutritional Tip: Make it a meal with a glass of your favorite juice, no sugar added. It is easy to prepare in just 15 minutes.

Ingredients:

4 cups of fruits, fresh and/or canned no sugar added: blueberries, mango, apples, bananas, pineapple, grapes and oranges.
1 small package (3 ½ ounces) of pudding mix of your choice
1 ¾ cups of milk (use nonfat or 1%)

Directions:

1. Make sure that you rinse the fruits and cut them into little pieces.
2. If you use canned fruits, open the can and drain the liquid.
3. In a bowl, add milk, pudding mix of your choice, it can be vanilla or lemon, mix it well.
4. Add fruit pieces over the pudding and mix well.
5. Let it stand for 15 or 20 minutes in the refrigerator.
6. Save the rest in the refrigerator.

Nutritional Information:

Per serving: 110 calories, 2 g protein, 24 g carbohydrates, 0.5 g fat, 170 mg sodium

7 Day Sample Menu Plan

Based on a 2000 calories/day diet

We all know how hard it is getting the hang of a new diet, especially one such as the Dash diet. Offered below is a seven day sample menu plan so that participants can get an overall idea of the different foods that you can have. Some recipes are included, they are marked by the symbol: *.

You have the flexibility to choose a plan according to your needs.

You can choose a diet anywhere from 1500- 3000 calories per day.

You can choose 1500 mg or 2300 mg of sodium per day.

The internet has a lot of resources and ideas for you to create the menu plan with the food that you most like. Check the resources area at the end of this book for a list of websites.

Day 1

Breakfast

Vegetable omelet: 297 calories
1 slice of whole wheat bread: 100 calories
*Refreshing Fruit Salad: 110 calories

Total calories for breakfast: 507 calories

Lunch

3 oz. of tilapia fillet: 268 calories
2 cups of green salad: 40 calories
1 slice of whole wheat bread: 100 calories
8 oz. of lemonade: 34 calories

Total calories for lunch: 442 calories

Snack

1 cup of orange juice: 111 calories
1 cup of low fat yogurt: 154 calories

Total calories for snack: 265 calories

Dinner

*Turkey Loaf: 150 calories
1 cup of garden salad: 20 calories
1 cup of asparagus: 27 calories
1 cup of nonfat milk: 87 calories
1 apple: 116 calories

Total calories for dinner: 400 calories

Dessert

1 banana: 105 calories
½ cup of low fat cottage cheese: 90 calories

Total calories for dessert: 195 calories

Total calories for the day: 1809 calories

Day 2

Breakfast

1 cup of nonfat yogurt: 174 calories
1 cup of fresh strawberries: 49 calories
1 boiled egg: 110 calories

Total calories for breakfast: 333 calories

Lunch

*Chicken with Oranges and Avocado: 366 calories
1 slice whole wheat bread with soft margarine: 200 calories

Total calories for lunch: 566 calories

Snack

2 slices of whole wheat bread: 200 calories
2 tbsp. of peanut butter: 188 calories

Total calories for snack: 388 calories

Dinner

1 cup of cooked lentils: 210 calories
1 cup of carrots: 25 calories
1 cup of mixed green salad (lettuce, tomato, carrots and mushrooms): 50 calories
1 tablespoon of Valley Ranch Salad dressing: 73 calories

Total calories for dinner: 358 calories

Dessert

*Baked Bananas: 310 calories

Total calories for dessert: 310 calories

Total calories for the day: 1955 calories

Day 3

Breakfast

*Applesauce French Toast: 150 calories
1 cup of nonfat milk: 87 calories

Total calories for breakfast: 237 calories

Lunch

6 oz. of salmon in orange grove juice: 517 calories
1 cup of cooked green beans: 44 calories
Total calories for lunch: 561 calories

Snack

1 slice of whole wheat bread: 200 calories
2 cups of papaya: 67 calories

Total calories for snack: 267 calories

Dinner

2 baked potato with the skin: 440 calories
1 cup of cooked carrot: 70 calories
2 cups of mixed green salad (mixed greens, tomatoes, cucumbers, red bell pepper and mushrooms): 100 calories
1 tablespoon of olive oil: 120 calories
1 cup of grapes: 106 calories

Total calories for dinner: 836 calories

Dessert

1 cup of nonfat milk: 87 calories

Total calories for dessert: 87 calories

Total calories for the day: 1988 calories

Day 4

Breakfast

Fruit cocktail:
1 cup of papaya: 55 calories
1 cup of strawberries: 53 calories
1 cup of watermelon: 85 calories
1 cup of grapes: 62 calories

Total calories for breakfast: 255 calories

Lunch

* Pear, turkey and cheese sandwich: 150 calories
1 cup of mixed salad (lettuce, cabbage, tomatoes and carrots): 50 calories
1 tablespoon of olive oil: 120 calories

Total calories for lunch: 320 calories

Snack

1 cup of nonfat plain yogurt: 154 calories
5 dates: 123 calories

Total calories for snack: 277 calories

Dinner

*Classic Grilled Salmon with Dill Sauce: 218 calories

1 cup of brown rice: 210 calories
1 cup of mixed salad (lettuce, tomatoes, carrots, mushrooms): 50 calories
1 tablespoon of olive oil: 120 calories

Total calories for dinner: 598 calories

Dessert

1 banana: 105 calories
1 cup of fresh squeezed orange juice: 112 calories

Total calories for dessert: 217 calories

Total calories for the day: 1667 calories

Day 5

Breakfast

*Oatmeal Waffles/or pancakes: 340 calories
1 cup of skim milk: 86 calories
1 cup of grapes: 62 calories

Total calories for breakfast: 488 calories

Lunch

3 oz. of beef steak: 214 calories
1 sweet potato: 180 calories
1 cup of green mixed salad (lettuce, tomatoes, carrots, mushrooms): 50 calories
1 cup of orange juice: 122 calories

Total calories for lunch: 566 calories

Snack

1 cup of celery: 20 calories
1 cup of carrots: 52 calories
2 tablespoon of Valley Ranch Dressing Salad: 146 calories

Total calories for snack: 218 calories

Dinner

3 oz. of turkey breast (without skin): 161 calories
1 corn tortilla with low fat cheddar cheese: 100 calories
1 banana: 105 calories

Total calories for dinner: 366 calories

Dessert

*Yogurt, Blueberries, Almonds and Honey: 200 calories

Total calories for dessert: 200 calories

Total calories for the day: 1838 calories

Day 6

Breakfast

1 cup of nonfat yogurt: 174 calories
2 cups of fresh strawberries: 98 calories

Total calories for breakfast: 272 calories

Lunch

1 piece of chicken casserole: 662 calories
1 cup of green salad: 20 calories

Total calories for lunch: 682 calories

Snack

1 cup of apple juice: 113 calories
1 slice of whole wheat bread: 100 calories

Total calories for snack: 213 calories

Dinner

*Chicken and Vegetables Stir Fry: 340 calories
1 cup of watermelon juice: 70 calories

Total calories for dinner: 410 calories

Dessert

1 cup of cantaloupe melon: 186 calories
1 cup of water melon juice: 70 calories

Total calories for dessert: 256 calories

Total calories for the day: 1833 calories

Day 7

Breakfast

*Peanut Butter & Banana Smoothie: 285 calories
*Vegetables and Cheese Egg Muffin Omelets: 104 calories

Total calories for breakfast: 389 calories

Lunch

*Non Mayo Tuna Salad: 245 calories
1 slice whole wheat bread: 120 calories
1 cup of orange juice: 112 calories

Total calories for lunch: 477 calories

Snack

2 tbsp. of peanut butter: 188 calories
1 cup celery sticks: 25 calories

Total calories for snack: 213 calories

Dinner

2 cups of fish soup with vegetables: 312 calories
1 whole pita bread: 140 calories
1 cup of honeydew: 50 calories

Total calories for dinner: 502 calories

Dessert

1 cup of fresh strawberries: 49 calories
15 almonds: 170 calories

Total calories for dessert: 219 calories

Total calories for the day: 1800 calories

Tips for Success on the Dash Diet

You have taken the first step in bettering yourself and have started the Dash diet. It is a little overwhelming how much dedication and self-control it takes to maintain a diet. You might find yourself slipping on and off the wagon at the beginning. You are worried that you might not have what it takes to keep up with this diet. Never fear, the tips for success are right here.

Take it Day by Day

Rome was not built in a day so you should not believe that your dieting success will start from day one. It is almost impossible to start a successful diet right off the bat no matter who you are. The best way to ease into a diet is to start small and gradually ease into it until the diet is just another part of your life. You should start by including a few dash diet meals into your routine. This could be three meals a week until you feel comfortable and able to move up until all your meals meet the requirements for the Dash diet. If you wake up one day and you just cannot go through the day without a slice of chocolate cake, eat the slice of cake. If you try to deny yourself your cravings, it could make it worse and you will run the risk of binge eating.

Menu Plans

Menu plans are your best friends when on a diet. Trying to choose a meal to cook when you are hungry is probably not the smartest thing to do while trying to adhere to a diet. When you make menu plans it eliminates the need to ponder around your kitchen, wondering what to make for dinner. You will have a seven day sample menu plan with a set list of the meals that you are going to make that you know will abide by the guidelines of the Dash diet. The Internet has a lot of resources and ideas for you to create the menu plan with the food that you most like.

Try a Different Variety

Food is not the enemy, this is a fact that most dieters tend to forget. Food can be your friend if you know how to give it a little variety. If you usually use whole milk in your coffee, next time you go to pour yourself a cup of coffee use the skim milk. Try some fat free yogurt with little slices of fruit in it for breakfast. Replace snack chips with fresh vegetables or fruit with a low fat dip. Try different herbs to flavor your meats and add a little more color to your plate with things such as carrots, eggplant, broccoli, and any other colorful fruit or vegetable that sticks to the Dash diet guidelines.

Portion Control

This is important for any successful diet. Portion control is probably one of the hardest parts to dieting. We don't think about how much food we actually put in our mouth during the day. When it comes to meal time we tend to eat the kind of things that we like and sometimes we might pile our plate a little too high. The self-control to not overload your plate with food is called portion control. It is a set amount or size of food that you are allowed to eat in order to stay healthy. Many people find that they gain weight because they don't know how much food is too much. With the Dash diet you will never have to worry about not knowing the right portion size.

Reduce Sodium

One of the biggest things about the Dash diet is that it cuts back on sodium and fats. While the Dash diet encourages a person to reduce sodium, it is not actually a requirement as long as you don't go over the set limit of sodium. The Dash diet standard for sodium is no more than 2,300 mg of sodium per day. However, if you reduce your intake of sodium to 1,500 mg of sodium per day you will see much better results.

Exercise

Exercise is fundamental in any diet. You should not expect to not work out and lose weight, it just does not work like that. Exercise does not have to be hard; you can incorporate exercise no matter where you are. If you know you are going to be in the office all day maybe you should consider investing in a pedometer. A pedometer is a little device that you hook to your person that tells you how many steps you took, and some models will tell you how many calories you have burned. You can even do simple things like dance a little while you are cleaning or go for short walks during your lunch break. Going for a walk during your lunch break comes with the added benefit of having more energy when you head back to work.

Water

Water is one of the best things for your body. It is also a good thing for diets. Water has no fats or calories, and it is the best way to rehydrate your body. Your body loses a lot of fluids a day and it is important that you keep hydrated so that your body can maintain health. Water can also fill you up, so when you find yourself wanting to overeat you can drink a glass of water instead and it will make your body feel fuller. Water is also great for keeping all your inner systems functioning such as your kidneys.

Take Dash with You Everywhere

Your diet does not end or pause when you walk out the door of your house. It is important that you figure out how to integrate the diet into your everyday life. If you are a snack time kind of person, take healthy Dash approved snacks such as nuts or fresh vegetables with you to work so you will steer away from those vending machines. Take your lunch to work with you so that you know what you have packed will meet all the Dash requirements.

It is still fine to go out with friends for a nice dinner. Just because you are on a diet does not mean you have to sacrifice going out with friends. When you are out for dinner with friends there are many things that you can do in order to make sure that you can still adhere to your diet:

Ask the waiter to let the cook know that you want your meal cooked with reduced salt or no salt at all.

- Opt for fruits or vegetables as appetizers.

- Limit the use of condiments like mustard, ketchup, or mayonnaise because these condiments are packed full of sodium.

- Skip the breads, skip the butter, and ask for low fat dressings.

- Remember that it is not mandatory to clean your plate. Portion control is key.

No matter the reasons why you decided to start dieting it is always possible to succeed.

Conclusion

Over the course of this book we have learned how the Dash diet, Dietary Approach to Stop Hypertension, can help you lower your blood pressure and your weight by following a few simple guidelines. We have discovered that one third of adults in America suffer from obesity and that it is a major cause of hypertension and heart diseases.

We have looked at an overview of the Dash study and learned that what started out as a simple idea quickly became something much more. The study's compelling conclusions started a revolutionary way to approach dieting and overall health. A diet had finally been found to have more concrete health benefits than most diets in the past.

We uncovered numerous more health benefits than just lowering blood pressure and obesity rates in America. We discovered evidence that the Dash diet can improve Type 2 diabetes by lowering levels in the same way that it works to lower high blood pressure. The Dash diet also works to increase a person's metabolism, and even helps with bone health. It lowers the risk of many life threatening diseases by changing a person's eating habits and sodium levels.

You were given the tools to get started. You were given equations to figure out where you are in your life right now. You learned that commitment and motivation were crucial in making the Dash diet work for you. You discovered that food was not the enemy and that you could still eat the foods you love, just in moderation.

You have been shown that exercise does not have to be menacing and can actually be fun. You have learned to keep positive and to remember that Rome was not built in a day, and that it is okay to stumble a little bit.

You have been given additional resources such as a seven day sample menu plan and recipes to help in your journey to success and a better you. Portion control was shown to be one of the biggest adjustments to dieting, and you were given tips to make this easier for you as the dieter.

You have been given the information to be able to go out and make informed decisions about what you are eating and how it will affect your body. You have made the commitment to start working towards a better you and you have finally taken the first steps.

Are you ready?

Bibliography

Clinic, M. (2013, May 15). *Nutrition and healthy eating*. Retrieved August 14, 2013, from Mayo Clinic: http://www.mayoclinic.com/health/dash-diet/HI00047

Dash Dieting Eating Plans. (2013). Retrieved August 16, 2013, from Nutritional Education Services Oregon Dairy Council : http://www.dashdietoregon.org/why/DASH-Evidence

Kelli Miller, L. C. (2008). *DASH Diet Improves Women's Heart Health*. Retrieved August 17, 2013, from WebMD Health News: http://www.webmd.com/heart-disease/news/20080414/dash-diet-improves-womens-heart-health

National Heart, L. a. (1998,2006). *National Institute of Health*. Retrieved August 16, 2013, from US Department of Health and Human Services: http://www.nhlbi.nih.gov/health/public/heart/hbp/dash/new_dash.pdf

Overweight and Obesity. (2012, August 13). Retrieved August 14, 2013, from Center for Disease Control and Prevention: http://www.cdc.gov/obesity/data/adult.html

John A. Tayek, M. (2002, February). *Is Weight Loss a Cure for Type 2 Diabetes?* Retrieved August 18, 2013, from American Diabetes Association: http://care.diabetesjournals.org/content/25/2/397.full#ref-list-1

What Is The DASH Diet? (2013, January 11). Retrieved August 14,

2013, from MNT, Medical News Today:
http://www.medicalnewstoday.com/articles/254836.php

Resources

http://www.dashdietoregon.org/
http://healthyeating.nhlbi.nih.gov/
www.dietaryguidelines.gov
http://www.nhlbi.nih.gov/guidelines/obesity/bmi_tbl.htm
http://www.nhlbi.nih.gov/health/prof/heart/other/chdblack/aa_
manual/session6.htm#serving
http://www.health.gov/dietaryguidelines/2015.asp
http://www.nih.gov/

Conversions:

[i]1 kilogram (kg) = 2.20462 pounds

[ii] 2.54 centimeter (cm) = 1 inch

Abbreviations:

[iii] Tsp. = teaspoon

[iv] Tbsp. = tablespoon

[v] Oz. = ounce

Made in the USA
San Bernardino, CA
10 December 2013